THE QUEEN'S UNIVERSITY OF BELFAST

Medicine and the Community

J. H. ELWOOD
Professor of Social and Preventive Medicine

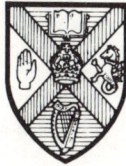

An Inaugural Lecture
delivered before the Queen's University of Belfast
on 27 February 1980

NEW LECTURE SERIES No. 121
ISBN 0 85389 180 X

Printed by
MAYNE, BOYD & SON, LTD, BELFAST

MEDICINE AND THE COMMUNITY

IT is a privilege for me today to give an Inaugural Lecture in accordance with the traditions of this university. My subject is *Medicine and the Community* and I intend firstly to outline some aspects of the development and teaching of Community Medicine at Queen's in particular, secondly to briefly describe some of my research interests and lastly to examine how community medicine may relate to the future provision of medical care and the improvement of the health of the population.

Community medicine derives from what the general public knows as public health. The term first came into use with the publication of the Report of the Royal Commission on Medical Education[1] in 1968 which was chaired by Lord Todd, Master of Christ's College, Cambridge. The Royal Commission defined community medicine as ' . . . the specialty practised by epidemiologists and by administrators of medical services, for example, medical officers of local authorities, central health or other government departments, hospital boards or industry . . . and by the staffs of the corresponding academic departments'. It is concerned not with the treatment of individual patients but with the broad questions of health and disease in particular geographical and occupational sections of the community and in the community at large. The essential difference between community medicine and clinical medicine as practised today is that community medicine aims at improving the state of the public health by developing and applying medical skills to whole communities rather than to individual patients. Because various terms such as state medicine, sanitary science, public health, social medicine, social and preventive medicine and community medicine have been used to identify this branch of knowledge I would like to place the development of this discipline at Queen's in the wider context of scientific public health as evolved elsewhere in the United Kingdom, Europe and North America.

The Public Health Movement

The founder of the public health movement, generally taken as spanning the period 1832-1854, was Edwin Chadwick[2] who was born on 24 January 1800 in the village of Longsight, near Manchester. He was by training a lawyer and was admitted to the Middle Temple in 1823[3]. His grandfather Andrew Chadwick, a staunch Methodist, founded the first

Sunday School in Lancashire and his father James Chadwick edited the *Manchester Gazette* and for a period the *Statesman* while its editor, David Lovell, was in prison. Edwin and his father were not very close and the latter emigrated to America in 1837. Edwin Chadwick is remembered by many for his report on *The Sanitary Conditions of the Labouring population in Great Britain* published in 1842 and by some for the acrimonious nature of his behaviour on committees particularly towards the end of his life when either he refused to attend meetings of the General Board of Health or else his fellow members refused to be present along with him. However, the Public Health Act of 1848 under which the General Board of Health was set up for an initial period of five years provided for the creation of local boards of health. Following the severe epidemic of cholera in 1848-1849 for which the Board was blamed, there was a strong demand for the appointment of whole-time Medical Officers of Health. The major epidemic of 1849 reached England via Hull with a case being diagnosed on board ship and it soon spread to other urban centres including Edinburgh, Leith, London and Glasgow. Andrew Malcolm, physician at the Belfast General (later Royal Victoria) Hospital, said the first case occurred in Belfast on 1 October 1849, the patient being in the Lunatic Asylum[4] which stood where the present Royal Hospitals are now situated. Henry MacCormac, who was the asylum's visiting physician at the time, does not mention this case according to H. G. Calwell's researches. However both Andrew Malcolm and Henry MacCormac agree that the later cases occurred in families who arrived in Belfast direct from Edinburgh and Glasgow. Eventually around 2 per cent of the population of Belfast was affected, some 2057 persons, and the mortality was estimated by Andrew Malcolm as 33 per cent. The first full-time Medical Officer of Health in England, William Duncan of Liverpool, was appointed in 1846 and the second, John Simon, became Medical Officer of Health of London in 1848 and later Chief Medical Officer to the Privy Council. By 1886 under section 21 of the Medical Act of that year, a Diploma or Degree of proficiency in State Medicine, Sanitary Science or Public Health became a registrable medical qualification and a pre-requisite for tenure of the post of Medical Officer of Health in the British Isles.

Sanitary Science and Public Health in Belfast and at Queen's
Belfast did not appoint a full-time Medical Officer of Health until 1890 but in 1849 six doctors[5] were appointed part-time 'Officers of Health' in the city among whom were Andrew Malcolm, the physician.

A second one was Samuel Browne[6], a consulting surgeon at the General Hospital, the Samaritan Hospital, attending surgeon at the Belfast Ophthalmic Hospital and in 1873 a member of the staff of the Royal Belfast Hospital for Sick Children. Samuel Browne as well as being the first ophthalmic specialist in Northern Ireland, later became part-time medical officer of health for Belfast, a post which he held until his death in 1890. Among many other offices he was Mayor of Belfast in 1870[7]. Another Belfast doctor who was greatly concerned with public health also was a well known surgeon. This was Henry "Health" O'Neill[8] who with his own money founded and published a journal called *Health* of which the first issue appeared in 1893. He crusaded not only for better sanitation and water supplies but also for improved factory conditions, better wages and control of drunkenness. The Diploma in Public Health or equivalent qualification was encompassed by legislation and is the only example in medicine of a degree or diploma required by statute for a particular medical specialist position. The universities had already recognised the importance of this subject and, for example, state medicine and sanitary science were acceptable for the Cambridge MD as early as 1868 and the DPH course started there in 1875[9]. In Ireland, William Stokes, Regius Professor of Physic in the University of Dublin advocated the importance of State Medicine[10] in his Presidential Address to the British Medical Association which was held in Dublin from 6-9 August 1867. A Diploma in State Medicine, the first of its type in this country was initiated at Trinity College in 1870[11]. By 1887 examinations for a Diploma in Sanitary Science were instigated by the Royal University of Ireland and these were held annually each June with papers in climatology, physics, sanitary engineering, hygiene, vital statistics and sanitary laws.

At Queen's, a part-time lectureship in Sanitary Science[12] was established in 1896 and held jointly by two lecturers, Edmund Albert Letts[13] from 1896-1909 and Henry Whitaker[14] from 1896-1906. Edmund Letts was born in Sydenham, Kent in 1852, educated at King's College, London, became Assistant in the Department of Chemistry at the University of Edinburgh and then Professor of Chemistry at University College Bristol from 1876-1879 before becoming Professor of Chemistry at Queen's from 1879-1917. He died one year after retirement in 1918 at Ventnor on the Isle of Wight. His colleague Henry Whitaker[15] was a graduate of the Royal University of Ireland. He was born in Belfast in 1833, entered Queen's College in 1854 and served an apprenticeship to become a licentiate apothecary in John Grattan's chemist shop in High

Street in 1856. Another apprentice at the same time was William Whitla who later became Professor of Materia Medica in 1890, was knighted in 1902 and on his death in December 1933 bequeathed his house *Lennoxvale* to the university as an official residence for the Vice-Chancellor. Henry Whitaker first qualified as a Licentiate of Apothecaries Hall, Dublin in 1856 and then as a Member of the Royal College of Surgeons of England in 1857 in which year he also obtained a Licentiate in Midwifery at the Coombe Lying-In Hospital, Dublin. He became an MD graduate of the Queen's University in Ireland in 1859 and received the Diploma in Public Health of the Royal College of Surgeons of Ireland in 1891. In addition he was a Councillor and later Alderman for St George's Ward from 1869 and was appointed the first full-time Medical Superintendent Officer of Health for Belfast in 1890.

What was Belfast like during this Victorian era? It was a rapidly growing industrial city, census enumerations of the population being for example, 52,287, 174,412 and 386,947 persons in 1831, 1871 and 1911 respectively. Some one in four of the working population were employed in the linen industry and ship building and engineering were equally important. The Belfast Rope-works virtually monopolized for a short time the market for binder twine in North America, the raw material being imported from Russia. This latter firm was founded by William Smiles, the son of Samuel Smiles[16] a medical graduate of Edinburgh and Leyden. William fathered eleven children, one of whom was Sir Walter Smiles who lived at Donaghadee and was a Member of Parliament at Westminster for many years until he drowned at sea within sight of his own home when the ship *Princess Victoria* sank on a crossing to Ireland in 1953. The products of the Belfast Rope-works were of such quality that the famous French tight-rope walker Blondin[17] crossed the Niagara Falls on a rope, 1100 feet long and 160 feet above the water, which was specially made for the occasion in Belfast[18]. Environmentally, Belfast was a dirty city with dust storms on windy days and street cleaning a rarity. Only a few streets in the centre of town were asphalted, the majority being laid with square sets of mourne granite. The road ended about the Botanic Gardens and from there was open country. Because of the rapidly growing population, there was an unceasing procession of carts bringing in bricks made from red clay in the neighbourhood and limestone from quarries in the Cave Hill. Stonemasons cut blocks of granite and sandstone in the streets while most of the timber arrived in sailing ships at the docks. Concerning health, the infant mortality rate in 1900 was 150 per 1000 livebirths[19], infectious diseases including typhoid and typhus fever, not to mention tuberculosis, dysentery and respiratory infections, were rife and the expectation of life at birth for baby boys was 47·1 years and for baby girls 46·7[20]. Scientifically there was progress on many fronts and much debate on Charles Darwin's book[21] *The Origin of Species* whose first edition was sold out on its publication day, 24 November 1859. Two debates on this issue are well remembered, the first being between Samuel Wilberforce, nicknamed Soapy Sam, the Bishop of Oxford who debated with Thomas Henry Huxley at the meeting of the British Association in that city on Saturday, 30 June 1860 and lost. The second is the address by John Tyndall[22], Professor of Natural Philosophy at the Royal Institiution which was delivered at the meeting of the British Association held in Belfast in 1874. These criticisms of the theory of evolution were reiterated in virtually every pulpit in Ulster.

The vacant lectureship in Sanitary Science 1906 was filled by William James Wilson for a period of three years and in 1909 he was appointed to a full-time lectureship in Hygiene. Also in 1909 the Diploma in Sanitary Science became the Diploma in Public Health. Dr Wilson held this post for twelve years from 1909-1921 when he became the first occupant of the Chair of Public Health at Queen's in 1921. On the establishment of this Chair the lectureship in Hygiene was discontinued. William James Wilson was born in 1879 at Straid Mills, Co. Antrim. He was educated at the Royal Academical Institution and at Queen's College Belfast from 1898-1906 graduating BA with first class honours in 1902, MB, with first class honours in 1905, MD with gold medal (the Royal University of Ireland) in 1907 and DSc (QUB) in 1910. He obtained the DPH from Cambridge University in 1906 and spent a short time studying at the University of Berlin. He held the Chair of Public Health[23] from 1921-1947, a period of 26 years during which time he combined his academic duties with appointments as bacteriologist and pathologist to the counties of Antrim, Down and Armagh and also as bacteriologist to the Belfast Water Commissioners. He published a book[24] entitled *Student's Textbook of Hygiene* in 1915 and conducted original research on the study and diagnosis of typhus fever and typhoid fever. His name is associated with a method of isolating and identifying the typhoid bacillus using the Wilson-Blair medium. He also developed an agglutinative method for diagnosing typhus fever which is known as the Wilson Weil Felix reaction, an acknowledgement[25] noted by the Queen's physician Sir Henry Tidy in his textbook of medicine. Tidy writes that priority for the principle of the test is due to James Wilson of

Belfast. This serological test is based on the observation that certain bacilli of the proteus group if isolated from the stools of typhus patients are agglutinated in high titre by serum of typhus patients. James Wilson published his findings in 1910[26] and restated them in 1917[27]. Much of the work on culturing bacteria and devising suitable media for their growth was carried out in association with Ethel Maud McVittie Blair who later was appointed to a lectureship in Public Health Chemistry in 1948. He served with distinction in the First World War as a major in the RAMC and in 1928 was elected Dean of the Faculty of Medicine, an office which he held until 1943. During this time the DPH course at Queen's was initiated. Professor Wilson died at his home, 10 Malone Road on 6 May 1954.

Public Health and Epidemiology in Great Britain and the United States

During the first half of this century public health at Queen's followed similar lines to the growth of this discipline elsewhere by initially being based on physical sciences such as chemistry and physics and on the principles of infectious disease control developed by the members of the Epidemiological Society of London which was founded in 1850 with the Earl of Shaftesbury as its first President. The sixteen medical scientists who worked with Sir John Simon in the medical department of the Privy Council brought the principles of the public health movement from theory into practice and also encompassed the new fields of bacteriology and pathology which were being developed. By the time of the First World War public health was being influenced by individuals in Europe and the United States as well as within the United Kingdom. Réné Sand founded the Belgium Social Medicine Association in 1912 and published an influential book entitled *The Advance of Social Medicine*. The Harvard School of Public Health opened its doors in 1922 mainly owing to the efforts of William T. Sedgwick, Professor of Biology and Public Health at the Massachusetts Institute of Technology. He is regarded as the father of academic public health in the United States and was a bacteriologist although he did not possess a medical qualification[28]. William Henry Welch at the age of 65 years resigned from his post of Dean of the School of Medicine to become the first Dean of the new Johns Hopkins School of Hygiene in 1918. William Welch[29], a bacteriologist and famous for discovering the bacillus which causes gas gangrene, now known as *Clostridium welchii*, designed a new type of curriculum in public health which included vital statistics and epidemiology. Wade Hampton Frost[30], born on 3 March 1880 in the village of Marshall near the Blue Ridge Mountains, joined the staff of the Johns Hopkins University School of Hygiene and Public Health in 1919 and became the first Professor of Epidemiology in 1927. One of his colleagues who joined at the same time and later became Professor and Head of the Department of Biostatistics in 1925 was Lowell J. Reed[31]. Welch persuaded John D. Rockefeller to donate substantial funds to public health and later served as a Director of the Rockefeller Foundation for several years. Meanwhile in Britain, London University had plans for the teaching of these subjects which resulted in the London School of Hygiene and Tropical Medicine offering its first DPH course in 1927.

Medicine between the wars in Britain is characterised particularly by the work of Sir Thomas Lewis who applied quantitative methods to medicine and developed what became known as clinical science[32]. He founded and edited a journal of the same name and did much to promote the clinical experiment as a means of understanding and interpreting signs and symptoms relating to patients and their illnesses. No examination of this era would be complete without reference to John Ryle. Ryle was a brilliant physician at Guy's Hospital who in 1935 became Regius Professor of Physic at Cambridge. He set up a university department of Clinical Medicine at Addenbrooke's Hospital but resigned from this prestigious chair to become the first Professor of Social Medicine at Oxford in 1943[33]. His influential book on *The Natural History of Disease*[34] is an important landmark in the development of preventive medicine. He died on 27 February 1950 of coronary thrombosis at the age of 61 years. By the Second World War, the public health movement's aims of reducing the toll of mortality from infectious diseases and increasing the expectation of life at birth had been largely accomplished, although certain major problems particularly the control of virus diseases such as poliomyelitis had yet to be solved. Attention was now turning to two important questions: could the methods used to clarify the epidemiology of infectious diseases be applied to non-infectious or non-communicable diseases such as coronary thrombosis, stroke, chronic bronchitis, cancer and accidents and secondly how best could current knowledge be applied in the form of a health service to care for the needs of the population? These objectives concerned the British Social Medicine movement and others from the 1930's onwards and are still major issues today.

Social and Preventive Medicine at Queen's

The Chair of Public Health was succeeded by a Chair of Social and

Preventive Medicine in 1948 and Alan Caruth Stevenson was appointed to the post that same year. Alan Stevenson[35] was born in Glasgow on 27 July 1909, educated at Glasgow Academy and the University of Glasgow from which he graduated BSc in 1930, MB in 1933 and MD in 1946. He was deputy Medical Officer of Health in Wakefield, Yorkshire and superintendent of the City of Wakefield Infectious Diseases Hospital prior to serving with the Royal Army Medical Corps during the Second World War. He attained the rank of colonel and served in Aldershot and with the 12th Army Corps in West Africa, and for a short time was deputy Director of Hygiene, Western Command. After the War he was Reader in Public Health at the London School of Hygiene and Tropical Medicine and Lecturer in Preventive Medicine at the Royal Free Hospital School of Medicine prior to coming to Belfast in 1948. His main interests were in the field of medical genetics, and the first genetic counselling clinic in Northern Ireland was set up under his aegis in conjunction with the Northern Ireland Hospitals Authority. He carried out distinguished work in relation to the cause of congenital malformations, associations between chromosomal aberrations and abortions and infertility, genetic causes of mental retardation, deafness and muscular dystrophy as well as estimating mutation rates for several mendelian inherited conditions including achondroplasia in the province. In 1958 Alan Stevenson was appointed to the directorship of the Medical Research Council's Population Genetics Unit at Heddington, Oxford, a post which he held until his retirement in 1973. He now resides in Inverness. Alan Stevenson's successor was John Pemberton who took up his appointment in 1958.

John Pemberton[36] was born in London in 1912, educated at Christ's Hospital School and studied medicine at University College London and University College Hospital, qualifying MB in 1936 and MD in 1940. He obtained a DPH from Leeds University in 1957 and was elected a Fellow of the Royal College of Physicians of London in 1964. He spent a period working at the Rowett Research Unit near Aberdeen under Lord Boyd Orr on the subject of nutritional deficiency; this also was the topic of his Doctor of Medicine thesis. He was medical tutor and medical first assistant at the Royal Hospital Sheffield, Senior Lecturer and later Reader in Social Medicine at the University of Sheffield prior to coming to Belfast. John Pemberton had many interests including the role of air pollution in producing chronic diseases of the chest. A major project initiated during his time in Belfast and still continuing is a large scale study of the flax and linen industries[37] which has shown that certain workers exposed to flax dust develop a disease of the lungs called byssinosis which previously had only been legally recognised in the cotton industry. As a result of this survey byssinosis is now a prescribed disease in flax workers with benefit to many affected individuals in our community. John Pemberton also did much to further the aims of social medicine. Together with a small number of colleagues he founded the Society for Social Medicine and the International Epidemiological Association, previously called the Epidemiological Corresponding Club. From these small beginnings both societies are now important professional bodies in this field of medicine. He was chairman of several official inquiries, a member of the Health Educational Council of England and Wales and wrote or edited several books including *Will Pickles of Wensleydale.* This is a description of the life-time's work of a family doctor[38] in the Yorkshire Dales and of epidemiological observations made in his practice among which is an account of Bornholm disease. John Pemberton now lives in Hathersage near Sheffield.

Another most distinguished member of the Department of Social and Preventive Medicine during this period, and who needs no introduction to this audience was Dr Peter Froggatt[39]. Peter Froggatt was educated at the Royal Belfast Academical Institution and the Royal School Armagh before entering Trinity College Dublin where he collected several undergraduate prizes before graduating BA in 1950, MB (with honours) in 1952 and MD in 1957. He then obtained the DPH from Queen's in 1966 and PhD degree in 1967. He was appointed to a Lectureship in Queen's in 1959, became Reader in 1965, Professor of Epidemiology in 1968 and was elected Dean of the Faculty of Medicine in 1971 succeeding Sir Henry Biggart. He was appointed President and Vice-Chancellor of Queen's from 1 October 1976 in succession to Sir Arthur Vick. Peter Froggatt has conducted important research in the fields of human genetics, epidemiology, occupational medicine and medical history and his work combines the interests initiated by both Alan Stevenson and John Pemberton.

The Professorships of Public Health, later renamed Social and Preventive Medicine have therefore been occupied by an Irishman, a Scot and an Englishman over a period of 55 years. Whether these changes in title, like British Railways being renamed 'British Rail' will result in a better service or even faster trains is open for debate.

Department of Community Medicine

The Department of Community Medicine has a wide variety of

interests. These include studies of risk factors associated with coronary heart disease and the role of coronary care units in treating patients with heart attacks, the relationships between hazards in the environment and disease as exemplified by air pollution and chronic bronchitis and dust concentrations in flax mills producing byssinosis in linen industry workers. We also are conducting surveys of the prevalence of alcoholism in Northern Ireland and epidemiological investigations of congenital malformations, mental retardation and associations between different types of maternal and child care and subsequent pregnancy outcome. My own research is mainly in the fields of occupational health and perinatal epidemiology. At first glance there seems to be little in common between these two aspects of medicine but if we are to have a fit working population, it seems obvious to start with as many fit and as few handicapped newborn infants as possible.

I will now briefly outline some of my research relating to physical and mental handicap in infants taking as an example the problems of congenital malformations of the central nervous system[40]. The great majority of infants born with these defects have either anencephalus or spina bifida. These occur in about equal numbers although rare abnormalities such as hydrocephalus are not uncommon. About 250 new born infants in Northern Ireland each year are affected by these conditions. Embryologically, they are due to primary non-closure of the neural tube so that failure of anterior fusion produces anencephalus and failure of posterior fusion causes spina bifida. As anencephalus is a severe abnormality of the brain, all affected infants are stillborn or die within two or three days of birth. Spina bifida is different because a varying proportion, currently about 40 per cent in Northern Ireland, survive beyond the first birthday although many have severe physical and mental handicaps. Historically, the study of these defects has been associated with genetic departments but this does not make them genetic diseases. It follows that the relative importance of genetic and environmental factors in the causation of spina bifida and other neural-tube defects is a major question. If the cause were wholly genetic we would expect the risk of Irish parents having an affected child to be roughly the same no matter where they lived. On the other hand, if factors in the environment influenced this risk, the likelihood of having an affected child would differ depending on the social conditions in which the parents lived and on whether they resided in Ireland or another country. It so happens that because of a natural experiment whereby large numbers of Irish people left their homeland around the time of the great famine, it is possible to

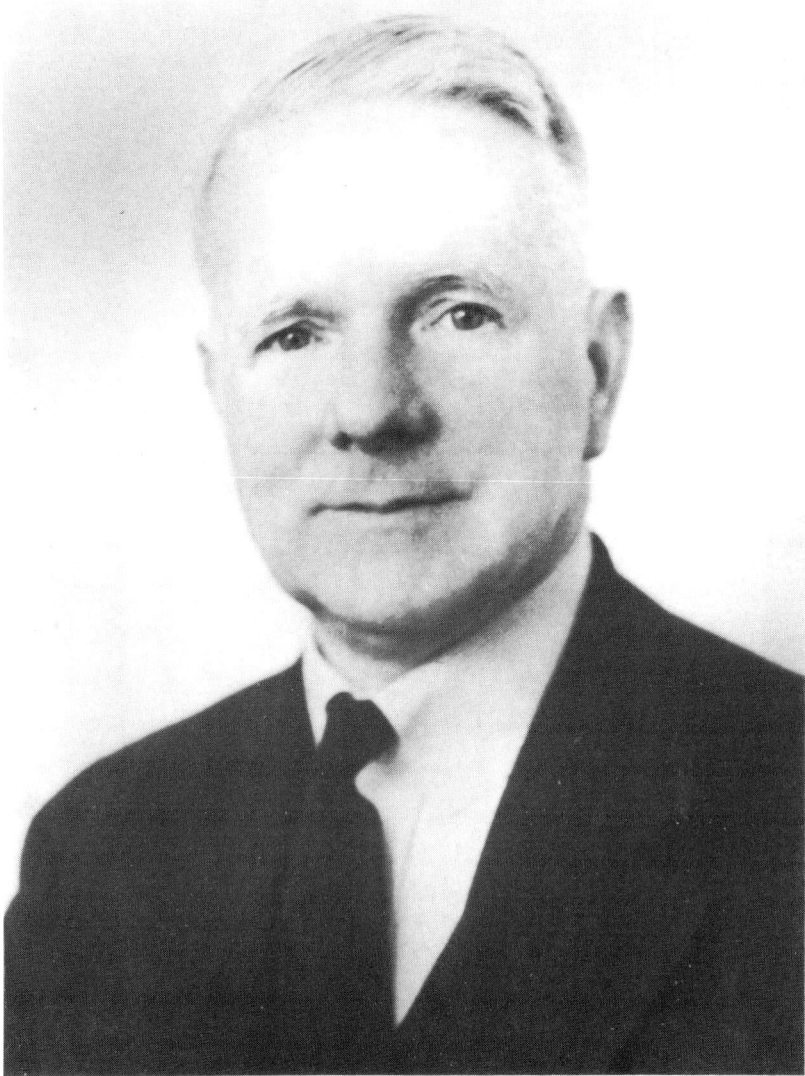

WILLIAM JAMES WILSON
Professor of Public Health 1921-1947

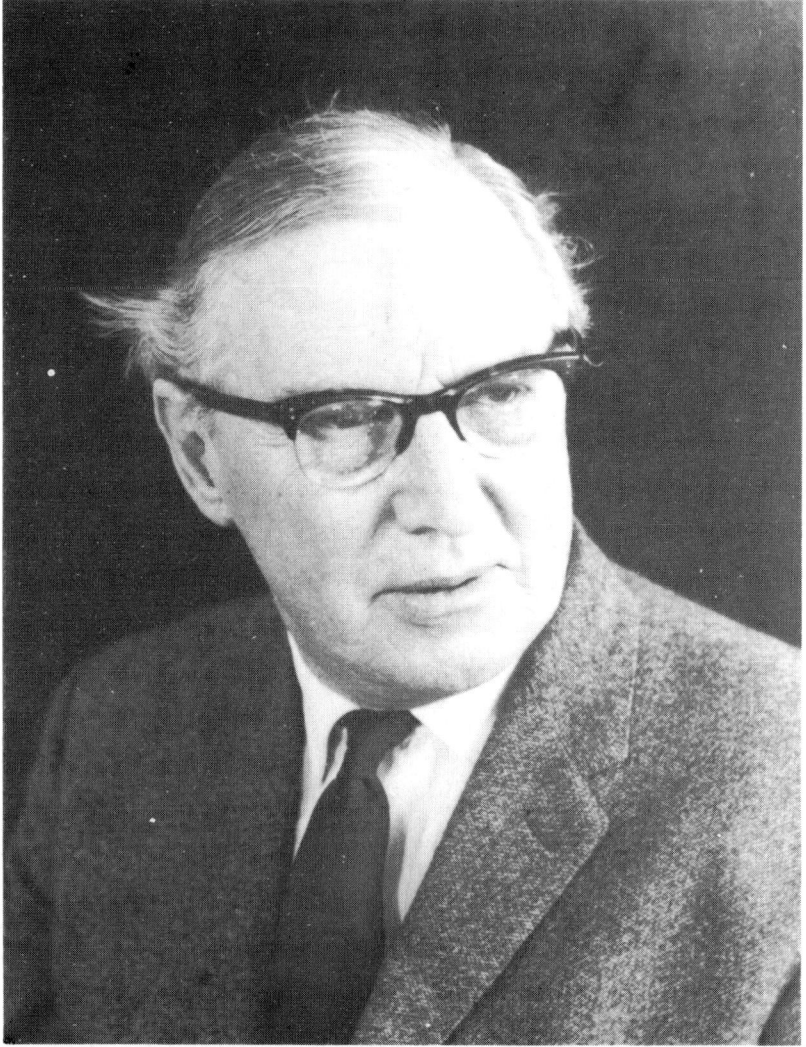

ALAN CARUTH STEVENSON
Professor of Social and Preventive Medicine 1948-1958

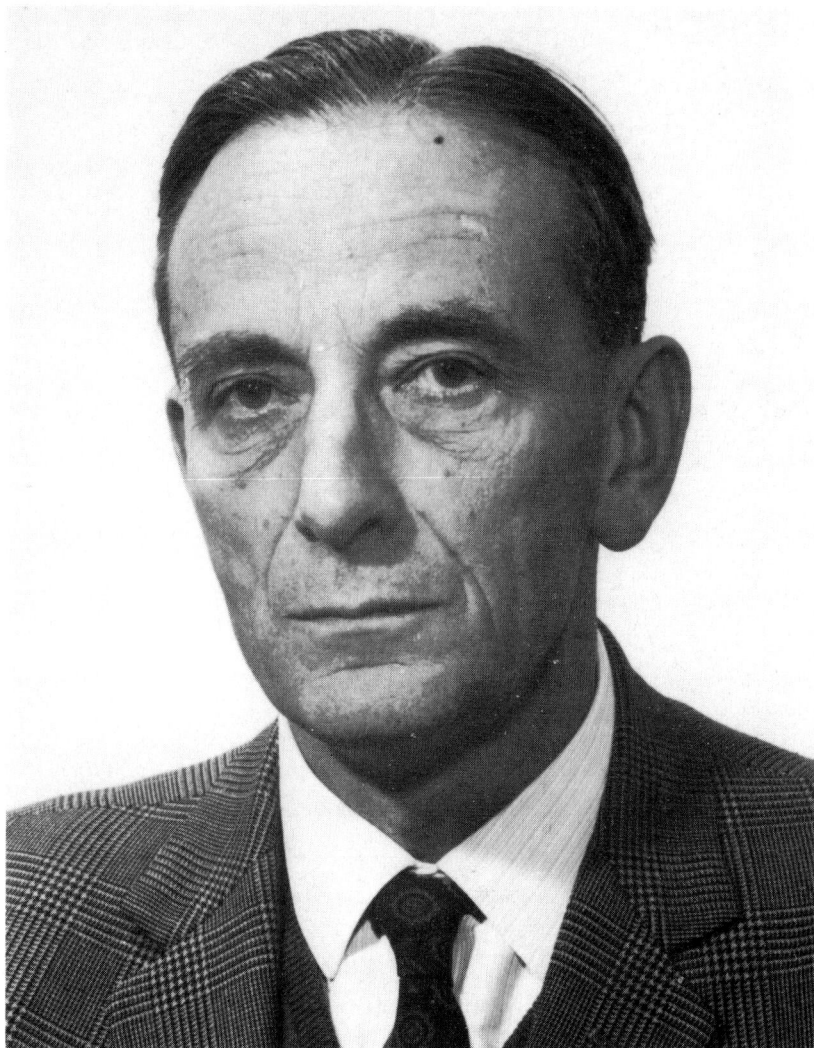

JOHN PEMBERTON
Professor of Social and Preventive Medicine 1958-1976

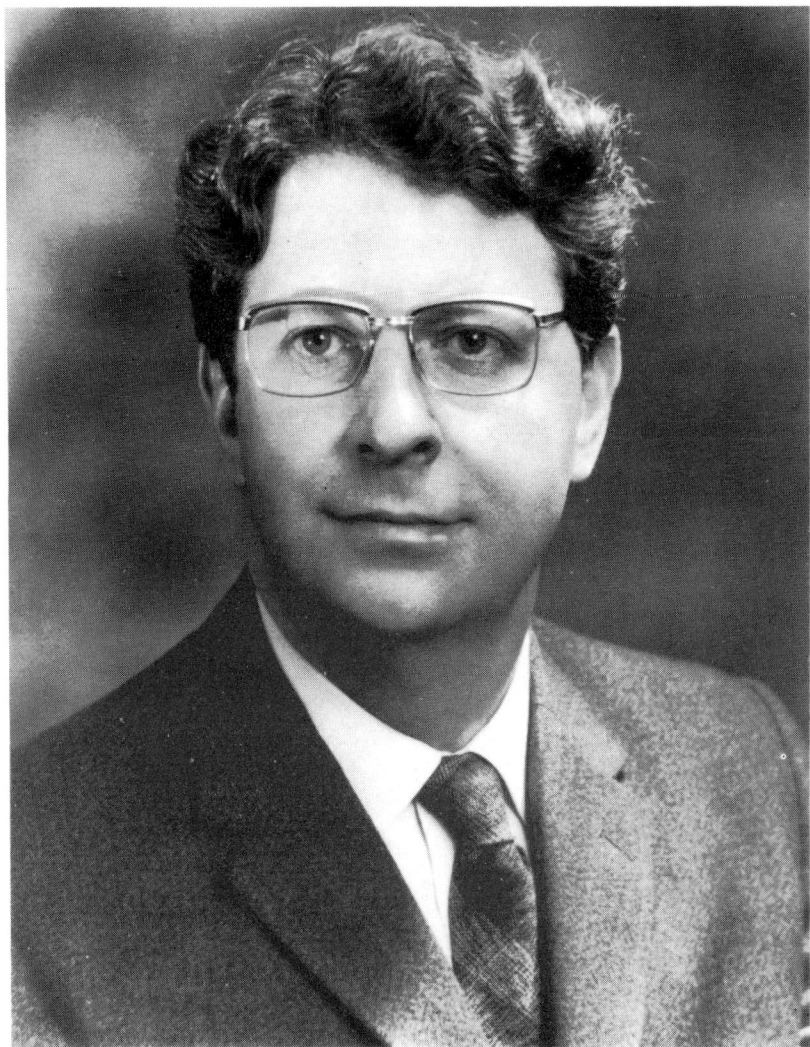

PETER FROGGATT
Professor of Epidemiology 1968-1976

test this genetic versus environmental hypothesis with reference to neural-tube defects. Today there are more persons of Irish descent living outside Ireland than within Ireland. For example at the 1841 census, 8,175,124 persons were enumerated but a decade later at the 1851 census there were 6,552,385 persons, a difference of over one and a half million and an annual loss of some 162,274 individuals. Of these one and a half million probably 50 per cent died because of the famine and accompanying disease during 1845-1849, whilst the remainder migrated with many going to North America. We therefore have a large community of Irish people resident outside Ireland and birth registers recording infants with congenital defects and parental ethnic origin are available in Boston, Massachusetts and in Canada. Birth registers also are available in Belfast and Dublin where virtually all infants born are to Irish parents. What do we find if we compare the prevalence rates of neural-tube defects in non-migrant and migrant communities?

TABLE I

Prevalence of Anencephalus at Birth by
maternal city of residence[40]

City	Rate*	Per Cent of Belfast Rate
Belfast	4·20	100
South Wales	3·09	74
Boston	0·98	23
Singapore	0·77	18
Melbourne	0·72	17
British Columbia	0·65	15
Paris	0·45	11
Sweden	0·37	9

*per 1000 (live and still) births

One of the first surveys of these defects was carried out in Belfast[41] by Alan Stevenson who found that the prevalence rates at birth appeared to be higher here than anywhere else in the world. Rates in Dublin are similarly high and it has now been confirmed that more infants with these conditions are born in Ireland than in any other country with nearly one out of every hundred births (live and still) being affected – (anencephalus 0·42 per cent, spina bifida 0·45 per cent, others 0·13 per cent). Comparable rates occur in South Wales but frequencies in Boston are only some 23 per cent of the Belfast figure while in British Columbia, Paris and Sweden the relevant proportions are 15 per cent, 11 per cent and 9 per cent respectively (Table 1). The most striking observation is that there are significantly lower rates in offspring of Irish parents living in Boston and Canada compared with the rates in infants born in Ireland. This applies whether the parents are rich or poor, Protestant or Roman Catholic. It is worth noting however in the Canadian data that the prevalence rates in the French Canadians and British Canadians are similar, despite the fact that frequencies in the United Kingdom are generally higher than in France. This was further investigated by examining a sample of 2352 control births and 796 cases of anencephalus born to mothers resident in fourteen Canadian cities. After adjusting for the confounding effects of ten other factors (year of birth, month of birth, maternal age, number of previous livebirths, stillbirths and child deaths, plurality of birth, legitimacy status, place of birth and city of residence) and comparing each ethnic group with the risk in offspring born to mothers of English and Welsh stock, only offspring to Russian or Oriental parents had significantly different and lower risks (Table II). Migration therefore of Irish mothers to North America substantially reduces the risk of malformation in their offspring; the Boston data also show that this risk continues to decrease in subsequent generations. If we look at longterm trends in the prevalence at birth of these defects the differences are even more striking. Since the Second World War frequencies of anencephalus and spina bifida have declined in Canada and Boston but have increased in Belfast and Dublin. Other differences in the epidemiology of these defects as observed in migrant and non-migrant Irish could be cited but the point I wish to demonstrate is that clearly factors in the environment are having a large effect on the numbers of such infants born in the community. It follows that if these factors can be identified and controlled, methods may be available which will prevent spina bifida and other malformations occurring. Unfortunately what these factors are is at present unknown. Many explanations have been put forward including dietary mechanisms such as ingesting blighted potatoes and folic acid deficiency, infections of the mother by influenza virus, rubella or other infections during early pregnancy or even in childhood or puberty. Hypotheses postulating tissue or cell interactions between foetuses in a multiple pregnancy or between an affected pregnancy and the remains of an earlier pregnancy

TABLE II

Risk of Anencephalus by Maternal Ethnic Origin
in Women resident in Canada[40]

Ethnic Origin	Adjusted Risk Ratio
England and Wales	1·00
Ireland	1·08
Scotland	1·04
France	1·01
Scandinavia	0·90
Russia	0·45*
Oriental	0·78*

*significantly different from the risk associated
with offspring of English and Welsh women

persisting in the wall of the uterus also have been examined. Furthermore, trace element deficiencies such as low levels of calcium or magnesium in drinking water or food have been suggested. Is the cause an unfortunate combination of an inborn error of metabolism in the mother relating to a substance essential for normal foetal development such as folic acid, and a relative dietary deficiency of this substance occurring at the time of neural-tube closure (around 28 days)? On the other hand, is the cause more complicated as for example a tissue reaction between two foetuses of what at the time of conception is a multiple pregnancy? According to this hypothesis, one foetus destroys the other and during this process, one foetus is absorbed or lost while the remaining continues to develop in utero but in a damaged condition. This damage is seen as a neurological malformation, the type and extent depending on the severity of the tissue reaction and its timing.

Community Medicine and Medical Care

This illustration of how epidemiology may clarify the possible cause of a condition such as spina bifida, once thought immune from external influence, is only one component of community medicine. Epidemiology, however, remains the scientific basis of this specialty. The other major component is how medical care should be provided for society and how the state of the public health can be improved. Since the era of

Sir Thomas Lewis, much progress has been made in evaluating medical treatments using retrospective, prospective and case-control studies as well as randomized clinical trials. Most doctors now accept that procedures and drugs should be tested for safety and efficacy prior to coming into general use or to replace existing therapy. However, the majority of the cost of the National Health Service is expended on care and not cure. Also, many ineffective therapies are still being used and effective therapies are being used inefficiently. The medical profession reacts strongly to allegations of prescribing useless treatments and yet these are offered daily by plumbers and car mechanics not to mention economists and politicians. Despite nearly a generation since the inception of the National Health Service, Dr Julian Hart[42] wrote in 1971 that 'the availability of good medical care tends to vary inversely with the need for it in the population served'. Currently, many assume that methods for evaluating the curative side of medicine cannot be applied or are irrelevant to the caring aspect of our profession. I would challenge this belief especially if present financial restrictions in the National Health Service are to continue for some time. If the 'cure' sector and pure research are to be stretched on the rack of the scientific method, the care sector, no matter how tender or loving, must be evaluated. Often a certain social or medical need is identified. However, before appointing a social worker or other person to meet this so-called need, we must evaluate evidence demonstrating that by providing an additional worker the natural course of the problem in question is significantly altered for the better; otherwise this is a complete waste of resources. Perhaps we can understand why some agree with Bernard Shaw who in the Preface to *Man and Superman* said 'Do not waste your time on social questions. What is the matter with the poor is poverty. What is the matter with the rich is uselessness'. Similar instances of waste of high technology medicine can be cited such as the availability of open heart surgery in eighteen London hospitals, all within a radius of ten miles of each other. Since reorganisation of the National Health Service in 1972 the situation has not noticeably improved and, if anything, curative medicine is becoming increasingly difficult to obtain. Waiting lists in the National Health Service are longer now than ever. Some 95 per cent of all admissions to the Royal Victoria Hospital currently are emergencies and even at the Royal Belfast Hospital for Sick Children the proportion is 45 per cent. What has happened to the idealism of the pioneers of the National Health Service who forecast diminishing demands for health care? Undoubtedly there has not been enough action in the field of preventive medicine and the situation has been likened to attempting to save an ever increasing number of people drowning in a river without anyone seriously questioning why they are falling into the water in the first place. I feel this is for two main reasons. Firstly, debate of these issues between the medical profession, the general public and politicians has been unequal, with politicians procrastinating and failing to act on the findings of medical research which would undoubtedly improve the state of the public health. Fluoridation of water supplies, stricter limitation and control of the use of tobacco, alcohol and drugs, rationalisation and better provision of obstetric and paediatric services are just some examples. Secondly, the model for understanding sickness and disease which assumes these problems may be investigated and controlled using the laws of the natural sciences such as physics and chemistry is now known to be incorrect.

Future Priorities

The Health Field concept described by Marc Lalonde[43] in the working document *A new perspective on the health of Canadians* or the Department of Health and Social Security's recent reassessment[44] of public and personal health entitled *Prevention and health – everybody's business* are perhaps nearer the truth. Let us examine the Canadian model as this was published before the British document. This identified four elements – human biology, environment, life style and health care organisation – as constituting an all-embracing Health Field concept. Human biology relates to the organic make-up of the individual, for example, the problems of understanding the genetic constitution, processes of ageing and the developing of chronic diseases. In the past millions of pounds have been spent on problems originating from human biology and many more millions have been devoted to health care organisation to the relative neglect of environment and life style. It was once possible to swim in the river Lagan but today if anyone is so foolish as to attempt this or rash enough to fall in he must be taken immediately to hospital to be de-infected. The river Blackstaff a tributary of the Lagan is the most heavily polluted river in the United Kingdom[45]. Do any of us believe that the millions of tons of raw sewage[46] that pass into the Lagan and the twenty-two million tons of raw sewage that pass into the Clyde each year do not constitute a health hazard?

However it is the life style aspect of health which probably will increasingly concern the medical profession in the future. A recent study by the medical services study group of the Royal College of Physicians of London[47] of the causes of death among 250 medical inpatients aged from 1 year to 50 years demonstrated a most disturbing finding. No fewer than 98 (39 per cent) of these individuals contributed to their own deaths by over-eating, drinking, smoking, not complying with medical treatment, refusing admission to hospital at an early stage of their illness or discharging themselves against medical advice once admitted. How are these examples of mass misbehaviour to be limited? The greatest progress in improving the health of the community in the future probably will occur because of changes in life style and environmental pollution control, although high technology medicine will play a part. These are not alternatives but must proceed in harmony. Devoting all our money to pure research and the efforts of the Medical Research Council in order to understand more about human biology by itself is not enough. Building more and more hospitals and tinkering with health care organisation by itself is not enough. Control of the environment by itself is not enough. Even so, what can one individual do if the water he drinks is contaminated with raw sewage so that he gets dysentery, if the house in which he lives has been built over an old chemical dump and his wife has a series of abortions or miscarriages and never bears a healthy living child, or if the food which he eats is contaminated by mercury and he develops mercury poisoning as has occurred in Minamata Bay, Japan and in the rivers of Northern Ontario? An eminent precursor of the importance of life style determining health is the poet William Wordsworth who lived for many years with his sister Dorothy at Dove Cottage in the Lake District. As Thomas McKeown, formerly Professor of Social Medicine at Birmingham University Medical School, points out[48] Wordsworth followed most of the rules of health now advocated by present day life stylists. He did not smoke or drink and unlike a number of his friends he did not dabble with drugs; in those days opium was in vogue. Wordsworth lived and worked in the open air, never became obese and walked about 180,000 miles during his life, an average of ten miles a day for sixty years – surely a daunting prospect for any aspirant jogger today!

Obviously no matter how good living and abstemious an individual may be there will always be sick people and therefore consideration of life style by itself is not enough. The message of Community Medicine for the future therefore is that we must have a much broader view of health and that all these aspects just mentioned must proceed together and should be provided with adequate resources. The reason why there should be greater resources devoted to prevention is not that economies will be produced in the National Health Service, as there is little evidence to support this idea. The reason is because prevention is more humane and will produce better health, resulting in less radical surgery, less ineffective medical treatment and ultimately true primary prevention of disease[49]. When James Wilson began his career at this university some 1 in 5 children died before their first birthday and 1 in 20 women died in childbirth. Infections were annual scourges in Belfast and killed many men, women and children, and diseases like typhoid fever killed thousands of soldiers in the trenches during the First World War where he served as a Medical Officer. When he retired the infant mortality rate was one quarter of the rate in 1900, death during childbirth was a rare event, and diseases like typhoid fever spread no further than two pages of a medical textbook. He saw the beginning of a National Health Service which has gone a long way to provide medical care for those in need, and the welfare services have virtually eliminated the great scourges of poverty and malnutrition. Progress throughout the rest of this century might not be as great or as striking as during the period that has passed but undoubtedly there will be progress if we extend our vision, particularly by facing up to the control of personal life style and of the increasing pollution of the environment. I mentioned earlier the great scientific interest aroused by Darwin's book *The Origin of Species* published in 1859, a subject still hotly debated and a topic reappraised on television and other media during the past year. The year 1859 also saw the publication of another book which since that date has sold millions of copies, has been translated into several foreign languages and yet is virtually unknown to the present generation. I refer to the book entitled *Self-Help* by Samuel Smiles[50], one of whose sons founded the Belfast Ropeworks. It is an interesting question whether students today would gain more by reading *Self-Help* than *The Origin of Species*. The relationship between health, work and life style described by Samuel Smiles, by the Hygieians of Ancient Greece, by Marc Lalonde in Canada or by the British Government in their recent consultative document is not new. They are however perhaps more relevant today when old lessons have to be applied to new and more complicated situations. What is the role of individual effort in a welfare state where social problems are supposed to be solved by government action? Why should we save in an economy where individual savings count for less and less every day and how can one man's efforts combat the problems of a collectivist environment? The community however is made up of individuals and health and welfare services do not eliminate or reduce the role of a single member of society. The medical profession never will be capable of curing all ills and we must recognise the importance of life style and factors in the environment which determine our health. If we wish to improve the state of the public health during the remainder of this century, in addition to clinical care provided by individual doctors, these other factors together with personal life style and the quality of our environment in particular must be evaluated and controlled. This should be the aim of the medical profession and the goal of every member of our community.

NOTES AND BIBLIOGRAPHY

1. Report of the Royal Commission on Medical Education Cmnd. 3569. HMSO, London (1968) para. 133.

2. Lewis, R. A., *Edwin Chadwick and the Public Health Movement 1832-1854*. Longmans, Green and Co., London (1952) p. 4.

3. Finer, S. E., *The Life and Times of Sir Edwin Chadwick*. Methuen and Co. Ltd., London (1952) p. 8.

4. Malcolm, A. G., *The History of the General Hospital Belfast and the other Medical Institutions of the Town*. (1851) p. 133. Reprinted in Calwell, H. G., *Andrew Malcolm of Belfast 1818-1856 Physician and Historian*. Brough Cox and Dunn Limited, Belfast, (1977).

5. Calwell, H. G., *The Life and Times of a Voluntary Hospital, The Royal Belfast Hospital for Sick Children 1873-1948*. Brough, Cox and Dunn Limited (1973) p. 12.

6. Calwell, H. G., *op. cit.* p. 12.

7. Owen, D. J., *History of Belfast*. W. & G. Baird Limited, Belfast (1921) p. 392.

8. Allison, R. S., *The Seeds of Time being a short history of the Belfast General and Royal Hospital 1850-1903*. Brough, Cox and Dunn Limited, Belfast (1972) p. 156-163.

9. Acheson, R. M. Medicine, the community and the university: a century of Cambridge history. *Br. med. J.*, **IV,** 1737-1741 (1978).

10. Stokes, W. President's Address delivered at the thirty-fifth annual meeting of the British Medical Association held in Dublin, August 6th, 7th, 8th and 9th, 1867. *Br. med. J.*, **1,** *101-102 (1867)*.

11. Widdess, J. D. H., *A History of the Royal College of Physicians of Ireland 1654-1963*. E. & S. Livingstone Limited, Edinburgh (1963) p. 181.

12. Moody, T. W. and Beckett, J. C., *Queen's, Belfast 1845-1949. The History of a University*. Published for the Queen's University of Belfast by Faber and Faber Limited, London (1959) Volume II, p. 656.

13. Moody, T. W. and Beckett, J. C., *op. cit.* p. 583.

14. Moody, T. W. and Beckett, J. C., *op. cit.* p. 657.

15. Whitaker, Henry. Obituary. *Br. med. J.* **I,** 1343 (1912).

16. Smiles, Aileen, *Samuel Smiles and his surroundings*. Robert Hale Limited, (1956) p. 25.

17. Blondin, real name Jean Francois Gravelet, was born at St Omer, France on 28th February 1824. He crossed Niagara Falls on a tight-rope several times in 1859, blindfold, in a sack, pushing a wheelbarrow, on stilts and carrying a man on his back. His last public appearance was in Belfast in 1896. He died in 1897.

18. Smiles, A. *op. cit.* p. 144.

19. Whitaker, H., *Report on the Health of the City of Belfast for the year 1900*. W. & G. Baird, Belfast (1900) p. 31.

20. Ulster Year Book 1975. HMSO Belfast (1975), Chapter 1.

21. Darwin, C., *The Origin of Species by means of natural selection, or the preservation of favoured races in the struggle for life*. First Edition. John Murray, London 1859.

22. Tyndall, J. *Address delivered before The British Association, Assembled at Belfast*. Longmans, Green and Co., London (1874) p. 1-65. Tyndall was born in County Carlow on August 2nd 1820 and died at Hindhead, Surrey, on December 4th 1893.

23. Moody and Beckett. *op. cit.* p. 657.

24. Wilson, W. J. *Student's Textbook of Hygiene*. William Heinemann, London (1915).

25. Tidy, H. L. (Sr). *A synopsis of Medicine*. Tenth Edition, John Wright and Sons Ltd., Bristol (1954) p. 296.

26. Wilson, W. J. The aetiology of typhus fever. *Journal of Hygiene, X, 155-176 (1910)*.

27. Wilson, W. J. Typhus fever and the so-called Weil-Felix reaction. (letter). *Br. med. J.,* **1,** *825-826 (1917).*

28. Acheson, R. M. Epidemiology and public health in American universities. (letter). *Br. med. J.,* **1,** *554. (1979).*

29. Burket, W. C. *Bibliography of William Henry Welch,MD, LLD.* The Johns Hopkins Press, Baltimore (1917).

30. Maxcy, Kenneth, F. (Editor). *Papers of Wade Hampton Frost, MD. A contribution to Epidemiological Method.* Oxford University Press and the Commonwealth Fund (1941) p. 3.

31. Maxcy, Kenneth F. *op. cit.* p. 12.

32. Booth, C. C. The development of clinical science in Britain. *Br. med. J.,* **1,** *1469-1473 (1979).*

33. Symonds, C. John Alfred Ryle. *Guy's Hospital Reports,* **99,** *209-229 (1950).*

34. Ryle, J. *The Natural History of Disease.* Second Edition. Oxford University Press, London (1948).

35. Queen's University Association annual record (1948) p. 21.

36. Queen's University Association annual record (1977) p. 64-66.

37. Carey, G. C. R., Elwood, P. C., McAuley, I. R., Merrett, J. D. and Pemberton, J. *Byssinosis in Flax workers in Northern Ireland* (1965). HMSO, Belfast.

38. Pemberton, J. *Will Pickles of Wensleydale.* First Edition. Geoffrey Bles, London (1970).

39. Queen's University Association annual record (1968) p. 29-30.

40. Elwood, J. M. and Elwood, J. H. *Epidemiology of anencephalus and spina bifida.* Oxford University Press, London (1980).

41. Stevenson, A. C. and Warnock, H. A. Observations on the results of pregnancies in women resident in Belfast. I. Data relating to all pregnancies ending in 1957. *Ann. Hum. Genet. Lond.* **23,** *382-94 (1959).*

42. Hart, J. T. The inverse care law. *Lancet, i, 405 (1971).*

43. Lalonde, M. *A new perspective on the Health of Canadians. A working document.* Information Canada, Ottawa (1975).

44. Department of Health and Social Security. *Prevention and Health everybody's business. A reassessment of public and personal health.* HMSO, London (1976).

45. Northern Ireland Council for Physical Recreation and Sports Council for Northern Ireland Joint Working Party. *The River Lagan.* Belfast (1979) p. 12.

46. Mellor, P. B. Samuel Smiles is Alive and Well. *Inaugural Lecture at the University of Bradford.* 3rd December 1974. p. 8.

47. Medical Services Study Group of the Royal College of Physicians of London. Deaths under 50. *Br. med. J.* **IV,** *1061-1062 (1978).*

48. McKeown, T. *The Role of medicine. Dream, mirage or nemesis?* Basil Blackwell, Oxford (1979) p. 111.

49. Cochrane, A. L. *Effectiveness and Efficiency. Random reflections on health services.* The Rock Carling Fellowship 1971. The Nuffield Provincial Hospitals Trust, London, (1972) p. 68.

50. Smiles, Samuel. *Self-Help.* Centenary Edition with an introduction by Professor A. S. A. Briggs (1958). John Murray, London. The first edition was published in 1859 by Dr Smiles at his own expense and risk. He kept the copyright and paid the publisher ten per cent commission. The manuscript had been rejected the previous year by Mr Routledge, owner of an established London publishing house.